PTSD

Pathways **T**hrough the **S**ecret **D**oor

by Timothy Kendrick

ISBN 978-1-4303-1319-9
Copyright 2007
LULU.COM

ABOUT THE AUTHOR

Timothy Kendrick is a retired Army Veteran who served in Panama, Somalia, Operation Iraqi Freedom and various other wonderful places in the world, Korea and Germany just to name a few.

He began as a military policeman with the 61st MP Company in the early 80's, switched to Combat Medic and then to Broadcast Journalism in the 90's when he was featured in Time Magazine (and several other media outlets) for his work in Somalia in 1993. His last Duty was in Iraq with the Department of Defense. He speaks five languages and currently lives in Tampa Florida.

Timothy (or Ty, as his army buddies know him) has traveled the globe five and one-half times and has dealt with his own PTSD. His motto is "It doesn't get any easier later, it just gets later."

DEDICATION

I wish to dedicate this book to several people who have given me inspiration during my struggles. My wife, Brenda, a.k.a. "Tutz" has stood by me through thick and thin. I cannot express in words how you have helped with your love and kindness. Behind every man, there is a great woman (with a boot at the backside when needed). Dr. Williams, for figuring out what was wrong with me; I cannot imagine what my life would be without his knowledge, expertise, and support. Dr. Milos Subervi who has been and still is a measuring stick for thoughts, my ideas, and me.

I wish to thank the many doctors that I educated through my insane behaviors, drunken binges, and bouts of rage including pride, lust, anger, greed, gluttony, envy, and sloth. We all learned something in the process over the past 15 years. I express my gratitude to every employer that fired me or that I told to "stick it." I learned burning bridges could be a positive motivating force.

Special thanks to my wrestling heroes who allowed me to live vicariously through them. It is truly "my soap opera." Linda and Vince

McMahan, who I have never met, but I learned how to turn "a negative into a positive" by there visions. You will never know what it meant to me to hear "Summer Slam" in Somalia in 1993 over the AFRTS radio live. Dusty Rhodes, "The American Dream," I learned it is okay to be different, thank you. Kevin Nash, who was always a shit to me when we were in Basic Training together but I knew you would be a star and set a standard somewhere, I always looked up to you. Not because of your height, because of your class, and the way you were then and have been throughout your career. The care you take in "keeping it real" and helping the young guys. Ric Flair, who proved there is no traffic along the extra mile. Bobo Brazil (RIP) when I was a kid, Ed Farhat, a.k.a. "The Sheik" (RIP) who would scare the crap out of the devil himself. I thank Jarrett promotions, for allowing me to be a ring announcer in 1986 for one special night in Clarksville Tennessee. To Bill Dundee for understanding that I knew how to "pay my respects" when I was in the locker room with the boys before the show. Hulk Hogan, or as dream calls you "yellow finger," at the old Cap Center in Landover Md. (I thought the ceiling was going to collapse circa 1985), there is no greater gift to give than to touch ones soul. That night like many others, you did just that. Rowdy Roddy Piper and anyone who has allowed "marks" like me to escape as we watched you in "the squared circle."

Tony Robbins, Wayne Dyer, Joseph Murphy, Brian Tracy, Tom Hopkins. Thank you.

My guardian angels "Delta Steve" in Mogadishu who I never met but I knew you were there, Also John Dahms in Mogadishu who taught me there is always a way from point A to Point B. David S. For pouring me on a chopper in Baghdad when "my glass was full." My Iraqi friends, who protected me, when I was in no condition to protect myself, thank you. Finally, Paul Miceli, a friend who is always there and has been through think and thin.. and think again

Many thanks to the enemy who for whatever reasons were lousy shots when it came to killing me (divine intervention). Thank you to the supreme creator of the universe. To the Universe for all the blessings that I receive on a daily basis.

PTSD
Pathways Through the Secret Door

Nights of the Werewolf

As I sit here and write this, I look back on 40 plus years of trying to figure out what was wrong with me. I will not remember everything due to over indulgence in medications. (Booze, pills, women and anything else I thought would fix me.)

My military life was very colorful, illustrious, for lack of a better term and very insane at times. I am getting a bit ahead of myself I suppose. I was born in an elevator in Holden, West Virginia. Talk about a dichotomy my childhood was up and down. My childhood was filled with the usual events of a child with divorced parents. I had massive mood swings from as far back as 4 or 5 years old. My heroes were sports figures, mostly professional wrestlers, and Evil Knievel. Evil was the epitome of "balls" when I was a kid. I use to jump trashcans on my bicycle pretending to be him.

In my mind, everything was black or white, no gray, no in between. It was all or nothing and that was how I lived from childhood until I was 38 years old. I feigned confidence, took risks that no one in his or her right mind would ever do. This is everything from the jumping of garbage cans to drinking whiskey until I became so drunk I had to hold onto the grass to keep from falling off the earth, and volunteered for every suicide mission I could go on in the Army. Rage was my constant friend and companion; I had no inkling of peace for many years. The only peace I had ever known was the adrenaline rush with the garbage cans, living in the doghouse (my fort and escape) and flying over and into combat with the military. (Facing death or ignorance)

I must tell you about the doghouse. My doghouse was a place I escaped to when I was a kid. I would sit in it for hours and dream of ways to make the doghouse fly away and take me to anywhere but there. I was too young to realize that if it did ever fly I still had to take "me" along. The irony of my "dog house" escape is; we did not have a dog; the previous owners left it.

I always felt like I did not fit in. It was like watching a movie, sometimes I was the leading character at other times I was sitting in the theater watching with my heart beating for fear of finding out the truth about me. The truth I might add that I did not even know at the time and the truth would get darker before it would get better. It would take me around the world several times because I despised "Garrison Duty" with all of its rules and regulations.

The title of this forward came about because of the nights I wake up and feel pain and indescribable fear all though my body. It reminds me of Lon Chaney Jr. in "The Werewolf." When I wake up at 2:30 or 3:00 a.m. and my body hurts and feels like a transformation of sorts. I go downstairs and huddle on the back porch away from the light that is over our pool. That is when I would turn into the Werewolf, my body aching, my mind racing 100 mph, trying to focus on anything but the fear and anxiety.

Sometimes I will see things that are not there, Or are they? Weird, other times the silence is deafening. In this book are some of my discoveries that have kept me from blowing my brains out, or destroying the ones I love. Thank you in advance for allowing me to share with you.

-Timothy Kendrick , SGT. U.S. Army, Retired

Sometimes in my bed at night
I curse the dark and I pray for the light
Sometimes, the lights no consolation

"Walking on a thin line" Huey Lewis

In this book, I will not go into details about the horrors of any war; instead, this book will show you how I fight the demons of Post Traumatic Stress Disorder. There is no sanity involved in it, because it affects each of us in a different way. The focus of this book is to express my viewpoints about what has kept me going in spite of having 28 jobs in 7 years. That last sentence shows that something was not right about me.

Most of us are bright, intelligent, and full of passion for a career that we believe in. The job choices we make, the spouse we choose, and the way we live our lives is a reflection of our primal positive instincts. Yet we jeopardize the things we love because of an emotional "anchor" or something that "triggers" our subconscious mind. Our conscious mind (ego) feels cheated or betrayed and we react on emotion. Emotion is what we are trained to act on when we were soldiers; we acted our way into right thinking. Now, we say things that we do not mean, quit our jobs, hit our boss, drink or use drugs ad infinitum.

Today, what keeps me at peace is "acting my way into right thinking." Motion creates emotion. We must do the things that will free us from our psychological slavery. I know this is easy to say, however massive action is the only thing that keeps me from just saying "what's the use" and digressing back into the darkness of my mind.

PTSD or post-traumatic stress disorder manifests itself in many ways. What I used to think had nothing to do with my anger, but had everything to do with it. Like the alcoholic, the drink is just the tip of the iceberg. The tip is not what sunk the Titanic. It was what was under the water that sunk the unsinkable, tons of frozen ice (your subconscious mind). I work daily on placing powerful positive messages into my subconscious mind.

Insanity is defined as "doing the same thing over and over, expecting a different result." I have stopped beating myself up about "good" or "bad" decisions because there are only "wise" and "unwise" decisions. The most important thing I can stress here is to act upon your decision. If it is not a wise decision, make another one. I have found that successful people make decisions swiftly and change them slowly. As a soldier, if you think through the actions that brought you to read this book (and survive) you will see on more than one occasion you had to make swift, quick decisions.

In war, there is no "paralysis by analysis." More so out here in the world striving to make a difference for our fellow man. What I am trying to say is do not over analyze anything. Make a decision, act on it, and if it is not a wise decision change it.

Beating yourself up over unwise decisions creates more havoc for you and the ones you love, it is like hitting yourself in the head with two hammers, when you use just one, feels pretty darn good.

LABELS

It seems society wants to attach labels to everyone. "He is Bi-Polar, a manic depressive, an alcoholic or he suffers from PTSD." These labels if accepted can inhibit or enlighten you, depending on how your process the labels. They can free you from your own self-limitations or you can allow them to strangle the life out of you.

I had heard all of the above labels many times. The one I never heard until I met a Doctor Williams from the 6th Medical Group was PTSD. I knew I was angry all the time, I knew my family walked on eggshells around me. I knew I could not keep a job. I had had a couple bouts of secret drinking. (My wife busted me; I lied by saying, "I only had two." What I did not tell her were the two I had included the first one and the last one, not the 14 or so in between).

Dr. Williams was brilliant because he took the time and saw something that every other Doctor had missed. When he explained what was going on in my head, he made drawings on the paper that covered the examination table. What he did was change my state, and break my pattern by writing on that paper while he explained how PTSD was affecting me.

A doctor may have said something to me about this before but I sure did not hear it until then, he got my attention, my wife and I were riveted. Dr. Williams did not just give me another label that I allowed someone to put on me it was a new door to open to my subconscious mind and a journey I will never regret. I finally had enough leverage and pain to make a decision and act on it.

INSPIRATIONAL DISSATISFACTION

I found the term "Inspirational Dissatisfaction" in a book somewhere and it states that when you have created enough pain in your life you will take the necessary action to change it. Sometimes it will be just a flash of inspiration such as writing this book after I walked off a 38k a year job and trying to figure out why. Granted 38k may not seem like a lot but I started at $10.50 an hour and in 3 years and several jobs later, I was at 38k. Inspirational dissatisfaction got me to that point.

The one truth I find in life is, by helping others we help ourselves. I am convinced this is the only way to gain any amount of peace or riches. Ask yourself, "What can I do to help someone else." While you are talking to yourself, ask what you really what out of life and most importantly ask yourself, "Why you want it."

A word of advice, do not expect any person who has never walked in a pair of combat boots to understand anything about your perception of the world or the things you have done. "Beware of wolves in sheep's clothing." Or even better "Do not cast your pearls before swine." In the "civilian" world I work in, making off the cuff remarks has landed me in more hot water (being fired or kicking someone's ass or mine being kicked) than I care to mention.

As soldiers we have lived life as only few can understand. "Been there, done that, bought the T-Shirt. We lived life, because we were so close to death.

Most of the people that I have dealt with are disillusioned with everything and are content to live in their misery. I chose to associate with these people. WHY? I chose these people because it was the easy road. I call it the four deadly D's, an endless cycle of misery.

THE DEADLY D'S
DENIAL-DELAY-DETOUR-DILEMMA

The first D is DENIAL, a favorite among many of us. We tell ourselves, there is no problem. Forget the fact, your family is scared to death of you, you cannot keep a job, and you drink like a fish. Let us not forget talking to dead people who might visit you. In our "perception," we say that "everything is alright" or "I'm fine." Fine acronym = F*d up, Insecure, Neurotic, Emotions.

The second D is DELAY. We say, "I have a problem, but I'll deal with it someday." SOMEDAY IS A ROAD THAT LEADS TO NOWHERE!

The third D is DETOUR. We make changes and convince ourselves that change will help. I will find a new gal or guy, that'll fix me or find a new job and drink only beer or perhaps use pills instead of booze or booze instead of pills." I am sure you have your own favorites.

The fourth D is DILEMMA. Whoever said, "The truth shall set you free" forgot to add "but first it will make you miserable as hell."

I am here to tell you that MISERY IS OPTIONAL! Remember that everything is a choice and the way we perceive things through our beliefs and values affects how we handle situations. How you see them is how you treat them and how you treat them is how they become. This includes the way you treat the person you see in the mirror.

If you hang around a barbershop, you will eventually get a haircut, an old saying but how true. Find positive people that will support you and stick with them. If we want to be successful, we must do what successful people do.

Change can happen in a split second. Change can create fear in our subconscious mind because most humans do not like change. Change can also make us rise above our current state of awareness and achieve things we never thought possible. On the other hand, we can allow change to cripple us psychologically so we may never take that next step that will free us from our negative habits and mindsets.

WHY WE FIGHT

First, we fight because we took an oath. Most importantly, we fight for our buddy next to us. Duty, Honor, Country, yes, ultimately it is for each other's survival.

From my experience in dealing with the VA (Veterans Administration) the only people who are going to fight any battles for you with them (and win) is AMVETS or the DAV. Do not attempt to get through the red tape and political bureaucracy of the VA by yourself. Let AMVETS or the DAV do it for you. The best part, it will not cost you a dime!

I finally went to see an AMVETS representative, he was gracious, helpful and did almost all of the paperwork for me (hell, I could hardly write my name). I received my compensation within 6 months. It would have taken the VA 3 or 4 years because of the backlog. The VA has assisted millions of returning veterans and I praise them for what they accomplish with their limited resources and funding.

If you were like me, you would keep putting off contacting the Veterans Administration until finally you gained enough leverage (pain) to take action. The VA much like our great countries political system has become a career for far too many who have far too little to offer. In all fairness, I have met angels and heroes at the VA that have passion for what they do by taking care of the great warriors who have served this nation.

I did go to a couple "Vet Centers" looking for help, but I did not find anything. You might, but I did not. It is not for everybody. In addition, AMVETS and the DAV can point you in the right direction with the VA as far as Vocational Rehabilitation and countless other benefits you have earned. Use whatever works for you. Alcoholics Anonymous is a great program also.

FEAR AND THE SUBCONSCIOUS

Fear can seem very real. It is our perceived value of fear that helps or hurts us while finding solutions to our daily challenges and problems. I believe that discourage is the opposite of courage. However, fear can cripple you to a point of not even moving or taking any action because of the unknown. Fear can take on a life of its own.   In combat, the Fear is indescribable.

What are we afraid of, fear of failure? Some of the great inventors and leaders of this world have failed before they found the solution they were looking for. Failing is not Failure, giving up is failure.

Are we afraid of success? I had to dig deep on this one because all of the unhealthy input I allowed put in my mind throughout the years. A poverty consciousness is very real.

Recently a man won $180 million in a Powerball lottery, today he is broke, his daughter committed suicide, and he filed bankruptcy. How might you ask? He had a poverty consciousness.

Wealth and riches will never be ours unless we change our perception of receiving and giving riches. Yes, giving them away. This is a proven fact, the Law of Attraction, and the Law of Nature that says the more you can give away to your fellow man the more you receive in return. What services can we render for our fellow man so we may have the "riches" that we desire for our families and ourselves?

My solution for fear is to take some kind of action. If that does not work, I take another action. Having walked where we have walked we know that motion creates emotion. When we move something happens to our physiological self and our mind becomes clear. It is what Tony Robbins calls "Changing Your State." Walk through your fear, though sometimes it is trudge through your fear. Either way you must get through it. Write it down, discuss it, and you will become stronger.

Think back to times when you overcame fears that were real. Think of successes that you had while overcoming those challenges and obstacles. If you have to go all the way, back and remember the odds of being born, as you swam through all of the other sperm cells to get to the egg. (I know this is weird) but you were the one who made it. You were the champion. Was that little cell, smaller than a pinhead afraid? Absolutely not! Find any challenges that you overcame in your past and put those back into your memory bank.

Remember that perception is reality to your subconscious. Your subconscious mind will take you wherever your conscious mind tells it to go. Your subconscious cannot distinguish between fact and fiction; it will only execute what it is told to do. This is why it is important to be careful what you put into your subconscious.

WRESTLING WITH PHYSIOLOGY

Anyone who knows me intimately knows that I have been a fan of Professional Wrestling all of my life. I love the storylines and the most exciting thing is watching a live event when there is no play-by-play announcer. The good guy comes to the ring, he is known as a "Baby Face." To me "Baby Face" represents my subconscious mind and he must conquer the "heel," or bad guy who represents my conscious mind.

The beauty of any match like this is the story telling that goes on with the physiology of the wrestlers' bodies. It does not matter if you are ringside or in the nosebleed seats, you will see how they communicate with their mannerisms to tell a story as the match goes on. (Motion creates Emotion)

Every night that they perform, they tell a story, entertaining the crowd, always the heel is whipping up on the baby face. The baby face has to come back; the heel continues to hammer him. It looks like the end is near and then "Baby Face" has a second burst of energy. But not enough, back down to the mat he goes (representing another failed attempt by the subconscious mind to break a pattern). The heel (conscious mind) tries to hold our hero down, the crowd is chanting for the baby face to get up, keep fighting. The baby face draws strength from his "mastermind alliance" (the crowd) to come back from the devastation of the heel and break the hold (your false beliefs) and he breaks the hold, the crowd is feeling the thrill. The baby face goes for his finishing move, clothesline, he springs off the ropes, and drops the knee. The official (the universe) counts the heel's shoulders to the mat 1-2-3. The baby face wins and the crowd goes wild. The goal is achieved and the reward is another victory for the subconscious. Why, because he did not quit.

Yes, you are probably saying, "wrestling is so F_ke" (I refuse to say that word or write it. Wrestlers cannot F_ke gravity anymore more than you can F_ke the law of attraction in the universe. If you feel it, if you believe it, you will, with enough leverage find a way to achieve it. Once again, surround yourself with people who support you and what you are trying to do.

Free yourself from the psychological chains that you have wrapped around yourself. You become your environment; attract to you the environment that you want.

Sadly, many wealthy athletes and performers can communicate with thousands of people every night but they cannot communicate with themselves. When this happens, they self-destruct. THIS IS FAILURE. You can have it all and if you do not learn to control your thoughts and emotions, you will die a thousand deaths. Feed your subconscious with powerful messages and more importantly take massive action toward a major definite purpose. Create within yourself a burning desire to continue through the challenges that come your way and will only make you stronger.

Remember:
Act Your Way into Right Thinking

THE PAST DOES NOT EQUAL THE FUTURE
Unless you choose to live there
-Tony Robbins

What do you think of when you think of courage? There are a million definitions because no two people perceive the same thing the same way. Everything we see, do, and say are based on our perceived beliefs and values.

What is the opposite of courage? I use to think it was fear, but it is not fear it is DISCOURAGE. I became discouraged and I became bitter, negative, my perception was skewed. To get from discourage back to courage you must encourage yourself (corny but true).

Think of an accomplishment that made you feel good. Relive that moment, think of any awards you received. It is important to stay focused on courage and away from fear. Wherever your focus is, that is where you will end up.

Insanity is defined as doing the same thing repeatedly but expecting a different result. Remember when we fall short of our goals we set for ourselves this is an opportunity to learn and try a new approach. This takes us back to courage. I call this (insanity) a "comfort zone" because you always know what you are going to get.

Comfort zones are like caves
Their darkness makes it hard to see
Their stagnant air grows stale and makes it hard to breathe

Their walls box us in
Their low ceilings keep us from stretching to our full height
                    -Jim Newman

Think of your journey out of this cave. The best way I have found is to visualize a ladder that I can climb. There is someone at the top reaching for my hand and I have my other hand behind me reaching down the ladder helping someone else. Napolean Hill says, "No man can become a permanent success without taking others along with him." Of the many jobs that I have had over the past 7 years, I learned one important thing that has kept me from falling completely in the gutter. Four magic words, "I need your help." Those four magic words have kept my ego in check, and helped me to help others. Who does not want to help someone when asked in this humble way? It is not pity; it is allowing someone to assist you.

You may think "I don't need anyone's help," but we do need others to help us. It is not what they can do for us, it is, what we can do for them. I have found that everyone wants, and needs to feel important. By helping others, we are helping ourselves and creating a bond with the universe. Remember what we put out is what we get back. If you need assistance, ask for it, you are not separate from your environment. Trust your inner self (gut) it has kept you going this long. I know it has taken me to a higher plane in spite of my personal defects.

THE RECKONING

General George. S. Patton stood on battlefields and said, "I've been here before." I understand what he meant. In Mogadishu and all over Somalia I felt it, I felt it in the Gulf, I felt it in Panama, and I felt it in Germany.

I used to think revenge meant redemption, now as I write this the word "reckoning" comes to mind. Hell, I am not even sure I know what that means

Dictionary.com defines it this way: v. reck ·oned, reck ·on ·ing,

Informal. To think or assume.

Phrasal Verbs
reckon with
> To take into account or deal with: a man to be reckoned with.

reckon without
> To fail to consider or deal with; ignore. I am still trying to figure out the previous page I wrote

To me "reckoning," means one must deal with a situation and bring it to its right place in the universe when in fact the universe is the way it is supposed to be (balanced). If you want to change anything in your life then make it "a must." The subconscious mind cannot tell the difference between what we have done and what we have created in our mind.

This being the case, I walk the thin line and make it into a two-lane highway by finding the truth or my version and perception of the truth. Perception is reality, this is very important in my life today. Thoughts are things.

GRATITUDE and ATTITUDE =

ABUNDANCE

I'M NOT A DOCTOR
...BUT I"LL TAKE A LOOK ANYWAY

Medication has always been an issue for me. I take medication only because I tried going without it and I destroyed everything that I touched. I almost lost my wife, isolated my kids and countless jobs (hell, my dog would not even come near me). I excelled at my jobs because I was always looking for the "rush" and used it to hide my secret. I made many people angry and burned every bridge I crossed so I could not return (sometimes, burning bridges can be a positive move).

I was flat broke and took a civilian job in Iraq (very smart with PTSD, let us go back to the party). I was totally insane and sacrificed my personal and physical well being for money. Lesson learned, I would never do that again.

This choice is entirely up to you, but (Beware Underlying Truth) if you did not go to medical school for 8 years I suggest you take counsel in what the professionals have to say.

You must find an outlet for your aggression. Like the alcoholic who cannot soberly analyze his destructive behavior, we cannot make ourselves aware of our own destructive behavior. I had a friend who tried to fill the void with booze and finally his ego and false pride would not let him hide any longer. It destroyed his family and finally it destroyed him with a gunshot to the head.

I have been hospitalized numerous times for various bouts of drinking, and flashbacks. I thought the drinking would make them go away, but it just made them worse. I kept my secret and it manifested itself outward in many forms like drinking, drugging, and promiscuity, just to mention a few. (Remember the 4 D's?)

Continually putting positive things into my mind every waking hour has saved me more times than not. My Doc says "I am functioning," I say to hell with that, I want to live like I'm dying, by remembering every second of every day and living in peace with myself and contributing to society. The past does not equal the future, today is the tomorrow you dreamt about yesterday.

FOCUS ON SOLUTIONS

I would like to tell you a great story about focusing on the solution instead of the problem.

This story is about a minister who on Saturday morning was trying to prepare a sermon under difficult conditions. It was a rainy day and his son was restless and bored. Finally, in desperation, the minister picked up an old magazine and thumbed through it until he came to a large brightly colored picture that showed a map of the world. He tore the page from the magazine ripped it into little bits and threw the scraps all in to the living room floor with the words:

"Johnny, if you can put this all together I'll give you a quarter." The preacher thought this would take Johnny most of the morning. However, within ten minutes there was a knock on his study door. It was his son with the completed puzzle. The minister was amazed to see Johnny finished so soon, with the pieces of paper arranged and the map of the world back in order.

"Son, how did you get that done so fast?" the preacher asked. "Oh said Johnny, "It was easy." On the other side, there was a picture of a man. I just put a piece of paper on the bottom, put the picture of the man together, put a piece of paper on the top, and then turned it over. I figured if I got the man right, the world would be right."

The minister smiled and handed his son a quarter. "And you've given me my sermon for tomorrow, too," he said. "If a man is right, his world will be right." If you are unhappy with your world and you want to change it, the place to start is with yourself. The solution lies within.

THE MAGNIFYING GLASS

Remember when you were a kid, and you found a magnifying glass in a box of Cracker Jacks? Well you held that magnifying glass in one place on a piece of paper and allowed the reflection of the sun to come through. The heat of the glass started a little spark that eventually became a small fire.

Well, your mind works the same way as the magnifying glass. "What you think about you bring about". When you focus with a burning desire upon your objective that tiny spark becomes a massive flame of achievement. You may not know this but a plane that takes off from Tampa, Florida flying to Atlanta Georgia is off course 95% percent of the time! How can this be you may ask? The answer is simply "The power of focus." The pilot knows his outcome Atlanta, he makes adjustments the same way you do when you drive a car.

The flip side is "what you resist persists." When you focus on a job you hate, or "the people that are out to get you" and not having enough abundance (look at these bills piling up?) Well, guess what? The resentment grows for the job, you send out hate, anger, and resentment to the people that "are out to get you" and the bills just snowball out of control. Your poor and false perceptions from your belief system become your reality.

The solution for me is gratitude. I can hear you groan as I write this. Gratitude, aagghh!!! "What you think about is what you THANK about, you bring about." This, I have found to be the greatest secret, THE LAW OF ATTRACTION. Remember, thoughts become things. You are the only one who creates your reality never forget this.

P S F
find the Problem; Solve it, and have Fun

Find the Problem, Solve it, and have Fun. Life is one shot. Dr. Wayne Dyer says, "If you knew who walked beside you every day you would never be afraid again." Do not ever say, "I'll laugh at this someday," why wait laugh at it now. Enjoy the journey, live in the now; look at what you can bring to the table. Receiving is contingent upon your generosity. Give, give, give, and you will receive in return.

I once read "Anger is a dubious luxury." Control your state and your emotions, one outburst of anger can destroy a beautiful day because it will snowball out of control.

The best advice I have received is from my brother Greg, he wrote it on the back of his senior picture he gave to me. It simply said, "Don't walk in my footsteps, walk over them, and make your own path." I still have that picture and have thought about that inscription over the years. Those were powerful words for an 18 year old to write to his younger brother. I stepped over his steps and made my own path, some wise and some unwise.

If you knew you could not fail, what would you do?

JOURNALING

I have notebooks filled with everything from profound revelations to plain gibberish. There is an old saying "the faintest ink is more powerful than the strongest memory." I read back through my journal and think "wow, what kind of an emotional state was I in when I wrote that."

Every night I make an effort to write down what I learned that day. I also write down my plans for the next day. I may not follow them to a "T" but I have cleared my mind of all the clutter and I sleep better knowing I have made some attempt at a plan of action.

Some of my scribbling is just numbers, names, goals, affirmations, and incantations. I even have a fine selection of cornball slogans (that have saved my life on more than one occasion). The most important thing is I am taking positive action. Remember when I write these down they burn into my subconscious. The subconscious as I have said before cannot distinguish between what is real or imagined. That last statement has helped me more than I would have ever imagined. I changed my beliefs and values about past situations. This allowed my healing to shift into autopilot.

Writing has made me push through different thresholds of stagnation. It allowed me to gain control of my emotional state. It is a MUST to be in charge of this wonderful mechanism called the subconscious mind. I have taken tragic events from the wars and turned them into positive living experiences. Willie Nelson said, "Everyone has their own snakes to kill." What may have destroyed me might not have even fazed you. This is why putting it on paper takes the fear out of it and puts it into a different perspective. Remember if we keep doing what we have always done, we will get what we always got (pain).

You can act your way into right thinking but one can never think their way into right acting. Look at the first three letters of the word ACTion? There is a story about two old crows sitting on a fence and one of them says to the other "I think I'm going to fly over and get some corn." How many crows are on the fence now? Two, because the one said, "I think." He never took action.

Action is the thing that makes your life plan become a reality. The crow had a plan, flying to get some corn but he never left the fence. Make a plan for the actions you want for the next day every night before you go to bed. This does two things, one it clears your head of an awful lot of what I call "Grand Central Station" thinking. Two, it gives you a plan of action to follow. The next day you may not get to every item you have on your list but this will keep you from sitting around all day like the crows on the fence and going insane. Sanity is defined as soundness of mind. With PTSD when we are alone we are not in very good company unless we are meditating or putting something positive into our subconscious, TAKING ACTION!

THE SOUNDTRACK IN YOUR MIND
The Emotional Jukebox

Someone once said that we all have a musical soundtrack that plays in our mind. Where did this come from? My guess is years of programming from everything from commercials to music. Everything we have ever seen or heard is in our brain somewhere. Have you ever wondered why a song is in your head and you cannot seem to get rid of it?

My research and questions to people have found that it may pertain to our emotional and psychological state at the time. I wake up and hear a song that may be a "trigger" or an "anchor" to something from my past. Sometimes it is about a girl, other times it will take me to places I do not wish to go.

Remembering things and forgetting them constitute two ways that our subconscious protects us. For some reason Veterans like us find ourselves vividly remembering incidents, people, places, and things that may have warped our thinking and judgment. Sometimes this will manifest itself negative ways, we may become isolated, have panic attacks or bouts of confusion. The practice that works for me is replacing those old songs with something new and different until I can handle them. Sometimes it takes leverage (pain) to take action on these situations. If we are in enough pain, we will respond with whatever action is needed for change to take place.

Create new memories with these songs or replace the words with something that makes you feel good. My neighbor burns his trash on his farm, I can smell it a mile away, and it takes me back to Somalia just about every time. Alternatively, another personal favorite of mine is when he shoots one of his cows in the head when he sells one. Just the gunshot makes my mind move into fight or flight mode. The other day I opened my truck door to let my dog out when we went to the park. Just the way the handle "popped" put a ringing in my ears and I was instantly back to a place I did not want to be. By practice, taking action and using trial and error I have learned to change my state in a split second and move to a more comfortable place.

I have become a firm believer in "garbage in, garbage out." I replace those songs (old ways of thinking) with other motivational material or with new songs (new ways of thinking) and I create a peaceful fun environment for my subconscious. Remember that our subconscious cannot distinguish between reality and fiction. It will only do what our conscious mind tells it to do.

If we say, "I can't" the conscious mind tells the subconscious "okay boys; he says he can't do it so let's prove him right." If we say, "I can" the conscious mind says "okay boys he says he can so let's make it happen."

THE NEXT RIGHT THING

Make decisions based on fairness to everyone, yourself included. Do what is right whenever possible. This will insure that your peace of mind is secure. Without peace, there is no success. There are no "good" or "bad" decisions, just "wise" and "unwise" decisions.

The most successful people act without hesitation (other than punching your boss in the mouth) when making a decision. These same individuals are slow to change that decision, but if the necessary result is not achieved, they will change their plan of action.

We learn from these decisions as we learn from people that we come in contact with, do not put off that task that will free you from the chains that bind you. At times that might be just getting out of bed. The world continues, change your state of mind. Remember, motion creates emotion. We want to achieve a *strong emotional state* because with this emotional state we can do whatever we choose to do, we can have whatever we desire when we live with a positive mental attitude. This attitude opens doors.

FAIL TO HONOR PEOPLE AND THEY FAIL TO HONOR YOU....
-unknown

Man have I had some jobs that were crappy. This is because of what I believed I was capable of doing at that time. All of the jobs that I chose, yes, I chose, were managed by exactly the kind of people I expected. At the one retail store I worked at I had a supervisor, she was just nasty and mean. Now I know she was just full of fear and I chose not to get angry and decided to see what I could learn from her. The above statement is what great lesson she taught me, *"Fail to honor people, and they fail to honor you..."* Then I told them "working here is like a monkey having sex with a porcupine, I haven't had all that I want but I damn sure had all I could stand." I handed her my keys and said, "It's been a pleasure."

You can learn from any situation in life. After I left that company, the other managers emailed each other things about me. They wrote that I had threatened people; I broke things, (shocking huh? PTSD), some of it may have been true. I know we have a capability to give people what I call "The Evil Eye" when we

47

are angry. I lost another job before that because I "threatened someone." I think that situation would have been until I told them, "I never said those things and if I decided to "cut their testicles off I would have done it not just talked about it." Not exactly "a massive action plan" for lasting success. I just kept at it, working on myself, knowing I had something to offer.

I began to ask myself better questions and I received better answers. I took responsibility for my actions and continued working on my state of mind. Stephen Covey says in his book "The 7 Habits of Highly Effective People," "Work diligently to understand than to be understood." This is how I found out I could learn more by listening to people than I could from talking. I think of it as a big spotlight and I keep the spotlight on the other person 80% of the time and on me 20% percent of the time. I just make sure I stay in healthy thriving environments. Remember, thinking does make it so.

NORMAL IS A SETTING
ON THE WASHING MACHINE

Here is a funny definition I found in some medical dictionary of PTSD. PTSD: A normal reaction to an abnormal situation. What? All I could think was "Normal" is a setting on a washing machine.

There is no normal for everyone, we are all different, and that is what makes us so unique. This is why we can help each other. This is one of the many secrets to life by helping others we help ourselves. Try not to speak ill of any man and do not judge others. Get all the facts you need to make your decision if something is right for you or not.

OLD PEOPLE ARE AWESOME

I remember meeting this taxi driver, he was like 89 years young, and I ask him, "Why do you do this?" After speaking with him I could tell he did not need the money. He said to me "If you stop you drop." Talk about changing my state. If you stop you drop, simply put, ACTION. This person wanted to contribute to his fellow man and he did and still does.

FINANCES

Financial trouble can ruin your relationships, cripple your judgment, and even destroy you emotionally and physically. There is a book called "The Richest Man in Babylon" (been to Babylon, weird huh) that will teach you the only truths about how to get ahead of your finances.

The basic formula states that no matter how many people you are in debt to, when you get paid ten pieces of silver, the first thing you do is take one piece of silver away for yourself BEFORE you pay any debts owed. Next you pay your bills, feed your family with the other nine pieces of silver. The secret is PAYING YOURSELF FIRST. Invest that one piece of silver or save it.

This has helped me with my psyche tremendously and assisted me when I have fallen short of a goal (like keeping a job.)

DEPRESSION

It takes so much energy to be depressed. You have to think negative thoughts, slump your shoulders, keep a frown on your face, and tell yourself that you are so unique because no one has your problems. Do not get me wrong depression is real and can paralyze you and you may need treatment with medications. However, much of the time we just need to GET OFF THE CROSS BECAUSE THE LUMBER IS NEEDED ELSEWHERE!

HAPPINESS

The happiest man is he who constantly brings forth and practices what is best in him. Happiness and virtues complement each other. The best people are not only the happiest, but the happiest people are usually the best at the art of living life successfully.
       -Dr. Joseph Murphy

Now Trudge Your Road to Happy Destiny

Conceive, Believe, Achieve
Wishing you happiness, joy, laughter, and prosperity in all that you do.

Email: rainmakerty@yahoo.com

OTHER HELPFUL TOOLS I HAVE LEARNED

Strengthen Relationships
Becoming a Friendlier Person

Do not criticize, condemn, or complain.
Give honest, sincere appreciation. Become genuinely interested in other people. Smile

Remember that a person's name is to that person the sweetest and most important sound in any language.

Be a good listener. Encourage others to talk about themselves. Talk in terms of the other person's interests. Make the other person feel important, and do it sincerely.

Gain Cooperation. Win people to your way of thinking To get the best of an argument - avoid it. Show respect for the other person's opinion.
Never tell a person he or she is wrong. If you are wrong, admit it quickly, emphatically. Begin in a friendly way.

Get the other person saying "Yes" immediately.

Let the other person do a great deal of the talking. Let the other person feel that idea is his or hers.

Try honestly to see things from the other person's point of view. Be sympathetic with the other person's ideas and desires. Appeal to their nobler motives. Dramatize your ideas. Throw down a challenge.

Be a Leader. Change Attitudes and Behaviors. Begin with praise and honest appreciation. Call attention to mistakes indirectly. Talk about your own mistakes before criticizing the other person. Ask questions instead of giving direct orders.

Let the other person save face. Praise the slightest improvement and praise every improvement. Be "hearty in your approbation and lavish in your praise." Give the other person a fine reputation to live up to. Use encouragement. Make the fault seem easy to correct. Make the other person happy about doing the thing you suggest.

Overcoming Worry
Fundamental Principles

Live in "day-tight compartments." (Chunk it down to smaller pieces)
How to face trouble: Ask yourself," What is the worst that can possibly happen?"
Prepare to accept the worst.
Try to improve on the worst.
Remind yourself of the exorbitant price you can pay for worry in terms of your health.

Analyzing Worry
Basic Techniques

Get all the facts.
Weigh all the facts - then come to a decision.
Once a decision is made, act!
Write out and answer the following questions
    What is the problem?
    What are the causes of the problem?
    What are the possible solutions?
    What is the best solution?

Break the Worry Habit

Keep busy.
Do not fuss about trifles.
Use the law of averages to outlaw your worries.
Cooperate with the inevitable.
Decide just how much anxiety something is worth and refuse to give it more.
Do not worry about the past.

Cultivate an Attitude for Peace and Happiness

Fill your mind with thoughts of peace, courage, health, and hope.
Never try to get even with your enemies.
Expect ingratitude.
Count your blessings, not your troubles.
Do not imitate others.
Try to profit from your losses.
Create happiness for others.Pray.

Don't Worry about Criticism

Remember that unjust criticism is often a disguised compliment.
Do the very best you can. Analyze your own mistakes and criticize yourself.

Prevent Fatigue and Worry

Rest before you get tired.

Learn to relax at your work.

If you run a household, protect your health and appearance by relaxing at home.

Apply these four good working habits:

When faced with a problem, solve it if you have the facts necessary to make a decision.

Learn to organize, deputize, and supervise.

Put enthusiasm into your work.

Do not worry about insomnia.

"A steady sea never made a skillful mariner."

HOW TO HAVE YOUR OWN MIND POWER

Author Nathan Blaszak has practiced and tested several techniques of mind power and shows the very best ways to make positive changes occur in anyone's life.

He tests and shares his breakthrough discoveries in surprisingly simple – to – understand format and his credibility is realized when you practice and use what he shows you. He may even also prove to become a valuable asset in your pursuit to happiness, money, power, love and prosperity… However, you have to make that decision. I will let you decide for yourself. Remember you can learn something from everybody.

What is Mind Power?

Unlike what others are teaching about mind power, real mind power comes when you have the ability to do whatever you want, when you want it, however you feel like doing it, and nothing can stop you. In reality, it is when you become successful.

Mind power is not wishing, willing, or imagining – it is "being."

If you could create your very own mind power technique that could lead you to infinite knowledge and genuine happiness, how would you do it? Is it possible to spread a belief automatically through your mind to eliminate the disease that clouds your judgment you may not even be aware of it?

Mind power has this idea built into it. It will spread beliefs around the deep recesses of your mind automatically from disease to disease, without you having to put much thought into it. One can also create beliefs to build positive results to occur as the power consistently continues to grow. This is the key aspect to mind power; it helps the individual and causes them to eliminate their weaknesses and move on to experiencing a more "lucky" life, once and for all.

For example, one type of "mind power technique" is a past time eliminator system. Many times you can use the past time eliminator system so you can free yourself from past pains that effect your present daily actions. This system begins to pick away through your past, chooses to confront these issues, one at a time, and then destroys their influence as it stores them somewhere else in your mind where their negative effects are no longer present.

The key to the reverse thinking system (another term for this technique) is you must take up the challenge to confront your fears and limiting beliefs and replace them with new ones. Only a few minutes a day to put forth your attention to what your mind provides for you to confront, as it locates these negatively planted seeds, is all that is required. I hope that you will begin to understand your real purpose and meaning in life and erase all your negative influences.

Here are few examples of possible mind power strategies:

Reverse Thinking: Your body cells record everything you experience even from the earliest moments of conception. The possibilities of having past memories that were painful are very high. This technique involves locating and recalling these experiences until all your past pains are confronted, understood, and eliminated. These past painful experiences are like a seed that grows into a web matrix of negative influences and limiting barriers that affect you and your circumstances, even right now. The goal is to reach your very first moment of pain. Once it is free, this matrix will collapse and your mind begins to function at its entirety and you become what are best described as "super being." Or simply put, having the ability to create your future and present circumstances as you see fit.

Positivism: This is simply the act of being positive and expecting positive outcomes to happen for you. Although, it is not much like what is commonly referred to today as positive thinking. It is much more than that. When you can learn to release a positivistic mind virus, it begins to build upon itself and lead you closer and closer to the reality you wish to live in. Alter a belief, and you can make whatever you desire come true for you.

The Universal Power: Learn to tap into the potent psychic power that is readily available to all conscious beings. Once discovered, this psychic power can attract to you what you desire, on demand, or if you wish, in the future.

I have never really seen anyone talk about this or go too much in depth about it.

Control: Understand how to control not only the reality that happens for you in the future and now.

Beliefs: - Ever wonder how some people just seem to get whatever they want and how they can get to be so lucky? Although they might not be aware, that they have but it is because they started their own positive mind virus. It is a simple yet extremely effective way to "hot wire" your brain into believing whatever you program it to believe. Moreover, it begins to grow and build upon itself as your desired future circumstances begin to manifest. If you can get your subconscious mind to "believe" certain things about yourself, you can make it true.

So what can these five techniques do for you?

Bring you money, your dream home, your dream career, the desired love of your dreams. Power, control… Everything you dream about having, that you have not yet gotten, but you can really have. You just have to have the right tools.

Mind power technology and development has been studied for years. Now, it is beginning to become a new science. Mind power is simply a formula that leads to new exciting realms of increasing the potential powers of your being that will bring about and make positive changes occur in anyone's life – including yours!

You never have to lose time or money on what does not work again. Having your own mind power can mean that every action you choose from now on can be a winner! The above sentence is a strong statement, isn't it? However, it is true. I almost surprised myself at just how powerful mind power techniques can be as I put mine in place. Every choice I made instantly became a winner...even when I lost and failed!

Let us say you place a belief in your mind and let it go to work for you, which takes you 5 – 10 minutes. You make choices then based on what you planted and what it provides. You start noticing that your course of action is leading towards what you desire to become.

You then feel prevented by a barrier and you realize that you must have made a programming mistake. Most people would call it a failure and allow themselves to be defeated by giving up before they even try. I use a different system, which reduces my risk of making mistakes. Instead of searching for generalized outcome, I program my mind to bring about a specific outcome. I first program my mind to bring to my awareness any negative barriers. My goal is to get this garbage out so I can move on to harvesting my dreams.

Using autopilot programming that automatically gives me the ability to set up a completely automated system to erase these past negative influences is where I started. Three, Seven, or even three hundred hours of confrontations can generate continuing relief of these influences. It may seem impossible, knowing that having to confront all these influences once to reap the rewards seems well worth the effort.

Instead of only having one shot to confront my first moment of pain, I have limitless tries to destroy them. Once they are destroyed, they are gone for good. Then I get to move on to demanding life to give me what I want without second questioning its ability to do so. Who do you think will produce more results?

My system actually goes one-step further. I always try to use an element of mind programming in the sense of eliminating the disease of the mind first. My favorite technique was reverse thinking* I am way past that stage now, but everyone must do this first.

By recalling the very first moment of pain or discomfort, I will give myself a chance to free my mind from this entire negative web matrix my mind has created over the years. This may require some effort to accomplish, but it can be used to produce more power and potential to achieve even my wildest dreams.

As my mind begins to break free from these influences and beliefs, I notice how my thinking capacity has increased and doors have opened before me that I never even knew existed. I seem to have started to inherit stronger intelligence and an excitement to live. I began to feel this mysterious sense of having felt this feeling before. Some time long ago.

There is no way I can begin to explain to you how I feel and just how incredible it feels to be alive. You just have to learn how to do start your own mind power and see for yourself.

I am talking about the exact process I went through that immediately changed my life and can begin to change yours too. Then, after you finish reading about and practicing the first part of your transformation, then you will have the option to take yourself up to an even higher level of awareness with even more mind power tools and techniques you can use to make life give you what you want.

Literally become the master of your own universe and forever use your amazing powers of the mind to increase your luck, happiness, wealth, and prosperity to bring yourself love, friends, admirers, as you thrive on the control and power you have learned to possess. Let us look at one of the major viruses that bring about very noticeable results and let us look at what happens when you do not have this mind virus working for you.

ERASE YOUR LIMITS AND BARRIERS & MOVE TOWARDS HAPPINESS FOREVER

Some people understand this concept... Others just do not get it Can you remember when you were young? I mean really young... like when your mother was still pregnant with you. The most common reaction I get to that question is "yeah right" or "I wouldn't want to remember." Well, I am here to tell you that you really can actually remember these times if you want to remember them. I call it reverse thinking. How does it work?

It is simple. To start this process, you have to understand what it would mean for you to confront these memories. You have already learned about the benefits you will get when you erase that very first painful mind seed that has been planted long ago in earlier chapters. Therefore, the next thing would be to start doing it. The process is simple:

Go to a place where you will not be interrupted and relax. Start focusing on your very first moment of pain or discomfort. It may help to affirm to yourself by saying out loud "I will now recall the first moment of pain or discomfort as it now can be located" If you're doing this correctly you should feel or hear your stomach growl (not because you're hungry) but because this energy is being brought out from deep within.

Then start to recall the experience. In your mind start asking this seed (as if you were communicating with it) questions. Ask what it can show you and why it is there. Ask if it is ready to come out and then ask why

As you ask these questions your subconscious mind begins to recall this very first moment of pain and reveals to you key factors that will bring you closer to releasing this negative energy. I have heard this technique referred to as "getting rid of the demon" only it is not mystical; there is a scientific explanation for this.

Your body and its cells record these moments of pain and hold this negative energy within, then link it to any outside influence. There it remains until confronted by your conscious mind and made understand that there is no reason these energies should be there anymore. These moments of pain could be causing you to run certain patterns in your life or cause you to believe something that is not true.

When I learned about this, it made me wonder just what it was that I had buried deep in my psyche. If there was a way that I could get rid of these automatic commands that have been lodged somewhere deep inside and break any pattern that I did not have any control of. I was amazed and surprised, or completely dumbfounded at what I had discovered. After recalling and replaying these automatic commands several times repeatedly, I finally began to release this energy.

I would cry, scream, yell... I would repeat phrases that clicked in my mind as to patterns that I have not realized I have been running in my life. I could not believe it but I believed the results. After about a month of confronting this "demon," I began to notice changes occur without even thinking about it. For instance, some situations that I would normally feel shy or hesitant were no longer evident. In fact, I surprised myself with my attitude and clarity of thought.

You will know when you use this reverse thinking method correctly, you will know it when you begin to feel free, and then even more free. Your thoughts become clear and certain negative emotions or barriers have vanished, and you find yourself surprisingly successful past your expectations and in ways you never even knew could exist for you. There is no way to determine how long it might take a person to erase all the negative thoughts but to spend a year to do it is time well spent. For some people it may take a couple of hours – everyone is different.

I am going to let you in on a little secret, if you succeed in getting rid of all your negative emotions from the past that are painful, you will automatically become rational and responsible. That means you will always do the right thing and there will be no such thing as dishonesty or irrationality for you. It would seem as though it never even existed.

You function and act exactly according to your nature, which is good, responsible, productive, everything positive. Observe a child that is learning how to speak. Watch how fast they can learn to talk and how incredibly honest and innocent they are. If you erase your first moment of pain, you will be just like that kid again. Lightning fast thinking that is not disrupted by dishonesty, laziness, or irrationality. As I said before, it will not exist in you. Your creativeness and pride level sky rocket.

Moreover, you think differently. Inside your mind, you become aware of all your perceptions at the same time. It will be as if you are in your own body, hearing, seeing, smelling, tasting, and touching at one time. You will think of your past memories that are only relevant to the situation you are in. You will be living in the NOW, now the past, not the future.

To transform yourself into releasing this incredible power is all that is required is for you to start confronting all your past negative experiences until you release their energy for good. You will know when you are doing it correctly because you will yawn, cough, gag, and even sometimes scream and cry until you make yourself sick. Good for you. The above statement may sound crazy but is better to take the time to allow this negative energy out rather than have it remain inside you?

Give your body some time to process and rid yourself of this energy, sessions every three days will provide recovery time. Some effects of this process may cause you to become a little ill. Make sure you drink plenty of fluids

(WATER) because your body may have to pass this negative garbage through and out of your body. That is another reason why waiting three days in between is a good idea.

You may also experience mood swings, but do not worry, they will not last (note from author: yeah like we have never experienced mood swings). It is a good sign to notice that your subconscious mind is processing and making sense of what you are releasing. The mood swings are a confirmation that you are making positive changes and adjusting to your newfound powers. I know it sounds crazy in parts but the idea is to rid ones self of self-defeating behaviors.

Here is an excerpt from one of my favorites authors
  --Dr. Robert Anthony

THE SECRET OF "DOING WITHOUT DOING"

By Robert Anthony, PhD

A common misconceptions most people operate under is that you get what you want in life by what you DO, or through the actions you take. Most believe that the DOING or action part is what makes things happen, not so, this causes you to create in reverse. Let me explain...

The reason we put a lot of emphasis on action is that we do not understand the power of our thought. If you analyze it, ninty percent of most people's actions are spent trying to compensate for inappropriate thought. The Chinese philosopher Lao-tsu said that, "In the practice of the Way, every day something is dropped. Less and less do you need to force things until finally you arrive at *non action*.When nothing is done, nothing is left undone". What he is talking about is "doing without doing"

The problem is that most of us are preoccupied with "doing." Unfortunately, most of our doing usually involves struggle. In the western world we are conditioned to be action-oriented, so we place a tremendous value on doing. We are so busy doing that we do not realize that all this "doingness" causes us to create in a reverse fashion.

Most of our actions are out of fear, worry or doubt because we believe nothing will be done unless we DO something. In other words, we are trying to force our desire into manifestation through action. If your decision to DO is dominant, then you will not focus on what you want to BE in the present moment. This causes you to mis-create because BEING is the first and most important step in the creative process.

Here is the secret:

It is not your action that makes things happen it is your intent. You can reduce the need for action to a very minimum by allowing yourself to focus on what you desire until you feel the positive energy begin to move within you. This energy is not based on doubt, fear, anxiety, worry, or need. If you focus on what you want instead of what you do not want, you will know when it is time to take action. When you do, it will be effortless. Doors open and the entire universe will conspire to assist you in your desire.

Put simply, you should take no action on anything until you have visualized your desire and made it real enough in your mind that your next action (step), whatever it is, seems like the most logical step. How can you know the next logical step? Here is the test that you can give to yourself before taking any action. If you focus on what you desire and still feel overwhelmed or anxious, then you are not ready for any action. You know you are ready when it feels like the next logical step is effortless. There is no effort, no strain, and no pain.

What we want to do is to use the leverage of energy, the same leverage of energy that creates everything in the universe. However, we are so caught up in the reality of WHAT IS, that we feel we must create everything through mental effort and physical activity.

Have you ever seen people who seem to have all the wonderful things in their life without much effort? It almost seems like they have an advantage over everyone else. Then you see the people who work the hardest usually have the least. That does not seem fair does it? Nevertheless, the universe works that way.

Unfortunately, those who work the hardest usually have the least because they have not learned the leverage of aligning their energy. They are going about creating their lives the hard way. They are trying to use their actions to create what they want.

We have been programmed to believe that in order to have what we desire we must work hard. How many times have you heard - "No pain, no gain?" The implication is that if you want to make something of yourself, you must work hard. The message is clear - if you are not hurting or struggling, you are not moving forward.

However, here is the truth - anytime you are struggling, you are mis-creating. Anytime you feel pain or struggle, your magnetic point of attraction is directed to that which you do not want, rather than to that which you desire. Read it again! Actions are necessary, but they are the last component of the creation processes. Actions cannot be used effectively to initiate results, because initiation is the function of BEING, then thought, then action.

Remember, the creation of anything is through your vibration. Everything vibrates, and it is by that vibration that we harmonize and attract experiences to ourselves. So before you act or do anything, first ask yourself, how am I vibrating? How do you tell? You tell by how you FEEL. Your feelings show you your vibration. How you feel determines what you attract.

When you use the process of creating by only focusing on what you want instead of what you don't want, you will see that the universe will provide a different set of circumstances for you that requires much less action. This puts you in a state of "doing without doing" or action without effort. Dr Robert Anthony Has Made A Life Changing Difference In The Lives Of Over 10 Million People Worldwide.

THE TOP 10 SECRETS FROM ANTHONY ROBBINS

Courtesy of Thomas Murrell, MBA CSP

1. YOUR POTENTIAL IS DETERMINED (OR LIMITED) BY YOUR SELF-BELIEF.

As the promotional material says the event was 'about creating breakthroughs, moving beyond fears and limiting beliefs, accomplishing goals and realizing true desires, turning dreams into reality, creating fulfilling relationships, and modeling the strategies of peak performers to produce a quantum difference in your life.'

If you cut out the hype, the simple message is if you believe in yourself enough you can achieve anything. A memorable one-liner was "the only thing that's keeping you from getting what you want is the story you keep telling yourself."

2. MOST PEOPLE HAVE SELF-DOUBT AROUND UNIVERSAL THEMES.

Ask anyone and most people will admit they lack confidence in some areas of their life. The interesting thing I learnt from this seminar is that this self-doubt is around universal themes. These themes cross age, gender, religious, cultural and language barriers. Common doubts include 'I am not good enough', 'I am lazy', and 'No-one loves me'.

3. YOU CAN LEARN MECHANISMS TO ELIMINATE SELF-DOUBT.

Robbins calls it 'immersion' where you break old patterns and build new ones by repetition. He uses many Neuro-Linguistic Programming techniques to achieve this with his audiences. He says, "Progress is not automatic."

A memorable moment in the seminar was when we had to visualize ourselves inside a bubble and inside that bubble was a series of videotapes neatly arranged in a time-line that represented all our memories in our lives so far. We had to pull out the negative videotapes and destroy them. This was followed by time spent visualizing the future and how your life will look 10 and 20 years from now.

4. BELIEF IMPACTS ON MANY LEVELS.

The Robbins message was that three things shape our self-belief. He calls them the Triad. These are our patterns of physiology, focus and language or meaning. He highlighted this with the quote: "where focus goes energy flows."

5. OUR VALUES AND BELIEFS SHAPE OUR ACTIONS.

Robbins believes you can "vanquish whatever is holding you back from taking action."

Walking barefoot across a bed of glowing coals is the physical metaphor he uses in his seminars to prove this point to the skeptics. Eliminate negative self-belief and take massive action is his keys to success.

6. TO CREATE POSITIVE OUTCOMES YOU MUST TAKE MASSIVE ACTION.

"Where focus goes energy flows" is a quote used by Robbins in his presentation to highlight why you need to know your outcome and why achieving this is a must.

Nevertheless, many people fail to take the next step. They delay, put off, and find many reasons or excuses not to act. Robbins believes "progress is not automatic" and "action is power." Take action, even if it is the wrong action. He says it is "never a failure if you learn something."

7. MATCHING & MIRRORING CREATES CONNECTION, TRUST & EMPATHY.

Robbins spent a fair amount of time in the seminar talking about and demonstrating interpersonal communication skills. He used people from the audience to show how the process of "matching and mirroring" the non-verbal communication and body language of others can be a very powerful way to connect with people. In essence, you create rapport by adopting the body language of the person with whom you are communicating. He believes "rapport is power" and "total responsiveness is created by a feeling of commonality." If you have learnt these techniques before and haven't used them for a while, I suggest it is time to dust them off and put them into action next time you are communicating with someone on a one-to-one basis.

8. ANYTHING IS POSSIBLE IF YOU FOCUS ON PASSION AND PURPOSE.

Robbins believes that "to have an extraordinary quality of life you need two skills: the science of achievement (the ability to take anything you envision and make it real) and the art of fulfillment (this allows you to enjoy every moment of it)." He says, "Success without fulfillment is failure." Find your passion and purpose in life. My purpose is to make a difference in people's lives and use my gift as a speaker.

9. MODEL YOURSELF ON OTHER ACHIEVERS.

To gain improvements quickly and step up to a new level of achievement, Robbins believes learning from others who are the best in their field is the fastest way to achieve success. He told the story of how he wanted to improve his tennis game and so employed Andre Agassi, the then number one ranked player to help him achieve this. Who could you model yourself after?

"People's lives are a direct reflection of the expectations of their peer group," according to Robbins.

10. SUCCESS IS BUILT ON A HEALTHY, HIGH ENERGY BODY, HEART AND MIND

If you are not healthy - all of the above points are a waste of time. Your health is determined and influenced by your lifestyle.

I had to add some "good" tools from folks who have had more years of studying human behavior than I have. When I started this journey, it took me an hour and a half to watch "60 Minutes" on TV.